The Complete Plant Based Diet Cookbook

Enjoy Your Meals

Thanks to These Recipes

Jason Noel

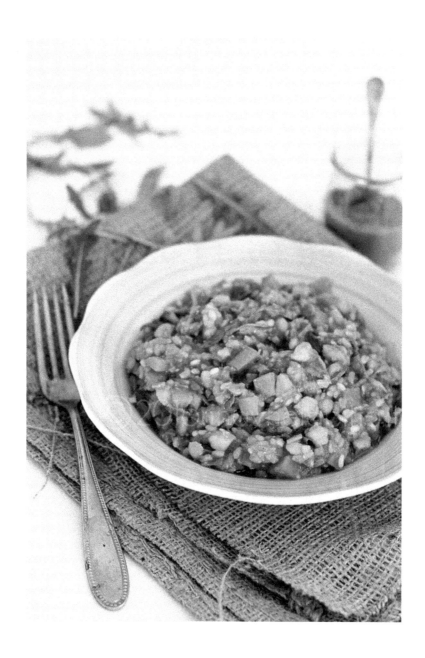

TABLE OF CONTENTS

Ginger Veggie Stir-Fry

Preparation Time: 10 minutes | Cooking Time: 15 minutes | Servings: 4

Ingredients:

- 1 tablespoon corn-starch
- 1 1/2 cloves garlic, crushed
- 2 teaspoons chopped fresh ginger root, divided
- 1/4 cup olive oil, divided
- 1 small head broccoli, cut into florets
- 3/4 cup julienned carrots
- 1/2 cup halved green beans
- ½ tablespoon soy sauce
- 2 1/2 tablespoons water
- 1/4 cup chopped onion

Directions:

• In a large bowl, blend corn-starch, garlic, 1 teaspoon ginger, and 2 tablespoons olive oil until corn-starch is dissolved. Mix in broccoli, carrots, and green beans, tossing to lightly coat.

• Heat the remaining 2 tablespoons oil in a large skillet or wok over medium heat. Cook vegetables in oil for 2 minutes, stirring constantly to prevent burning. Stir in soy sauce and water. Mix in onion and remaining 1 teaspoon ginger. Cook until vegetables are tender but still crisp.

Nutrition:

Calories 102 | Total Fat 8.5g | Saturated Fat 1.2g | Cholesterol 0mg | Sodium 91mg | Total Carbohydrate 6.5g | Dietary Fiber 1.6g | Total Sugars 1.9g | Protein 1.4g | Calcium 25mg | Iron 1mg | Potassium 154mg | Phosphorus 101mg

Roasted Green Beans

Preparation Time: 10 minutes | Cooking Time: 25 minutes | Servings: 4

Ingredients:

- 2 pounds fresh green beans, trimmed

- 1 tablespoon olive oil, or as needed

- Salt to taste

- 1/2 teaspoon freshly ground black pepper

Directions:

- Preheat the oven to 400 degrees F.

- Pat green beans dry with paper towels if necessary; spread onto a jelly roll pan. Drizzle with olive oil and sprinkle with salt and pepper. Use your fingers to coat beans evenly with olive oil and spread them out so they don't overlap.

- Roast in the preheated oven until beans are slightly shriveled and have brown spots, 20 to 25 minutes.

Nutrition:

Calories 48 | Total Fat 3.6g | Saturated Fat 0.5g | Cholesterol 0mg | Sodium 585mg | Total Carbohydrate 4.1g | Dietary Fiber 1.9g | Total Sugars 0.8g | Protein 1g | Calcium 22mg | Iron 1mg | Potassium 118mg | Phosphorus 91mg

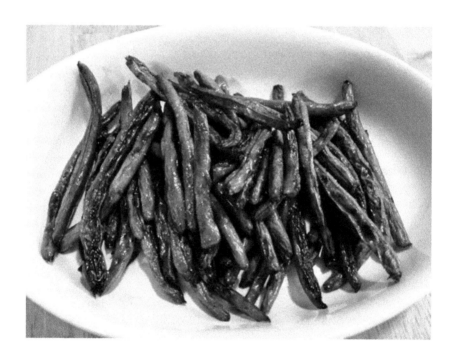

French Fries Made with Zucchini

Preparation Time: 10 minutes | Cooking Time: 25 minutes | Servings: 4

Ingredients:

- 2 medium zucchini
- 1 cup of soy milk
- 2 large eggs
- 3/4 cup corn-starch
- 3/4 cup dry unseasoned bread crumbs
- 3 teaspoons dried basil
- ½ cup olive oil

Directions:

• Peel and slice zucchini into 3/4-inch sticks, 4-inch long. Rinse zucchini and pat dry.

• In a medium bowl, mix milk and eggs until well blended. In a wide, shallow bowl, combine corn-starch, bread crumbs, and basil.

• Heat oil in a frying pan on high heat.

• Dip zucchini sticks into the egg mixture and then roll each piece in bread crumb mixture.

• Place in oil, flipping regularly, and fry for 3 minutes or until golden brown.

• Drain on paper towels and serve immediately.

Nutrition:

Calories 129 | Total Fat 11.7g | Saturated Fat 1.8g | Cholesterol 37mg | Sodium 44mg | Total Carbohydrate 4.6g | Dietary Fiber 0.5g | Total Sugars 1.6g | Protein 2.6g | Calcium 19mg | Iron 1mg | Potassium 109mg | Phosphorus 80mg

Garlicky Ginger Eggplant

Preparation Time: 10 minutes | Cooking Time: 00 minutes | Servings: 4

Ingredients:

- 2 cups eggplant

- 2 teaspoons minced ginger

- 2 garlic cloves

- 1/4 cup fresh Parsley

- 2 tablespoons olive oil

- 1/2 cup fresh mushroom pieces

- 1/4 teaspoon red chili pepper flakes

Directions:

• Slice eggplant into 1-1/2-inch-long pieces. Mince garlic cloves. Chop parsley.

• Heat olive oil in a large skillet. Add eggplant, ginger, garlic, and mushrooms. Stir-fry over medium-high heat until eggplant begins to soften, 4-6 minutes.

• Add parsley, chili pepper flakes to eggplant. Continue cooking for 1-2 minutes. Remove from heat and serve.

Nutrition:

Calories 78 | Total Fat 7.2g | Saturated Fat 1g | Cholesterol 0mg | Sodium 2mg | Total Carbohydrate 3.9g | Dietary Fiber 1.7g | Total Sugars 1.4g | Protein 0.9g | Calcium 10mg | Iron 1mg | Potassium 145mg | Phosphorus 48mg

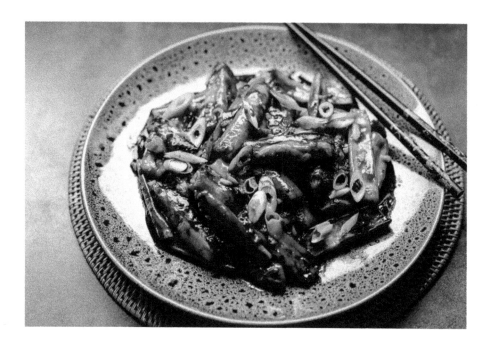

Garlic Kale Buckwheat

Preparation Time: 10 minutes | Cooking Time: 25 minutes | Servings: 4

Ingredients:

- 2/3 cup water

- 1/3 cup buckwheat

- 1 tablespoon olive oil

- 1 cup chopped kale

- 1 clove garlic, minced

- Salt and ground black pepper to taste

Directions:

• Bring 2/3 cup water and buckwheat to a boil in a saucepan. Reduce heat to medium-low, cover, and simmer until buckwheat is tender and water has been absorbed, 15 to 20 minutes.

• Heat olive oil in a skillet over medium heat; sauté kale and garlic in the hot oil until kale is wilted, about 5 minutes. Season with salt and pepper.

• Stir buckwheat into kale mixture; cook until flavors blend, about 5 more minutes. Add 1 tablespoon of water to the mixture to keep it from sticking.

Nutrition:

Calories 88 | Total Fat 4g | Saturated Fat 0.6g | Cholesterol 0mg | Sodium 9mg | Total Carbohydrate 12.1g | Dietary Fiber 1.7g | Total Sugars 0g | Protein 2.4g | Calcium 28mg | Iron 1mg | Potassium 151mg | Phosphorus 104mg

Glazed Zucchini

Preparation Time: 05 minutes | Cooking Time: 10 minutes | Servings: 4

Ingredients:

- 2 cups Zucchini

- 1 tablespoon honey

- 1 teaspoon corn-starch

- 1/8 teaspoon salt

- 1/4 teaspoon ground ginger

- 1/4 cup apple juice

- 2 tablespoons unsalted butter

Directions:

- Slice zucchini into -inch thick slices. Place zucchinis and 1/4 cup water in a pot. Cover and cook until slightly tender.

- Mix honey, corn-starch, salt, ginger, apple juice, and melted butter. Pour mixture over zucchini and water.

• Cook, stirring occasionally, for 10 minutes or until mixture thickens.

Nutrition:

Calories 86 | Total Fat 5.9g | Saturated Fat 3.7g | Cholesterol 15mg | Sodium 121mg | Total Carbohydrate 8.8g | Dietary Fiber 0.7g | Total Sugars 6.8g | Protein 0.8g | Calcium 12mg | Iron 0mg | Potassium 170mg | Phosphorus 56 Mg

Grilled Summer Squash

Preparation Time: 05 minutes | Cooking Time: 10 minutes | Servings: 4

Ingredients:

- 2 medium summer squash
- Non-stick cooking spray
- 1/4 teaspoon garlic powder
- 1/4 teaspoon black pepper

Directions:

- Wash summer squash with mild soap and water; rinse well.
- Cut each squash into four pieces; cut both vertically and horizontally.
- Place on a cookie sheet or large platter and spray with non-stick cooking spray.
- Sprinkle with garlic powder and black pepper, to taste (both optional).

• Cook on either a gas grill. Cook for approximately three to five minutes, flipping once. The squash should be tender but not mushy. If cooking on a gas grill, place the flat surface down on a sheet of aluminum foil sprayed with non-stick cooking spray.

• Cook approximately 5 to 7 minutes over a medium flame, watching carefully. Flip and cook for approximately 2 more minutes on the −round‖ side.

Nutrition:

Calories 17 | Total Fat 0.2g | Saturated Fat 0.1g | Cholesterol 0mg | Sodium 2mg | Total Carbohydrate 3.4g | Dietary Fiber 0.9g | Total Sugars 3g | Protein 0.9g | Calcium 18mg | Iron 0mg | Potassium 190mg | Phosphorus 100mg

Pineapple and Pepper Curry

Preparation Time: 05 minutes | Cooking Time: 15 minutes | Servings: 4

Ingredients:

- 2 cups green bell pepper
- 1/2 cup red onion
- 1 tablespoon cilantro
- 1 tablespoon ginger root
- 2 tablespoons olive oil
- 1/2 cup pineapple juice
- 1 teaspoon curry powder
- 1/2 tablespoon lemon juice

Directions:

- Chop bell pepper, onion, and cilantro. Shred ginger root.
- Heat oil and when hot add ginger and red onion. Cook until the onion is transparent.

• Microwave peppers on high for 6 minutes. Add the peppers to the onion mixture. Close the lid of the pan and cook on low for 10 minutes, stirring to avoid burning peppers.

• Add pineapple juice and simmer for 2 minutes. Add curry powder and cilantro. Turn the vegetables once and let simmer on low for 2 minutes.

• Garnish lemon juice before serving.

Nutrition:

Calories 107 | Total Fat 6g | Saturated Fat 0.8g | Cholesterol 0mg | Sodium 4mg | Total Carbohydrate 12.5g | Dietary Fiber 2.6g | Total Sugars 7.1g | Protein 2.3g | Calcium 20mg | Iron 1mg | Potassium 222mg | Phosphorus 150mg

Stuffed Mushrooms

Preparation Time: 25 minutes | Cooking Time: 20 minutes | Servings: 4

Ingredients:

• 8 whole fresh mushrooms

• ½ tablespoon olive oil

• ½ tablespoon minced garlic

• 1 (8 ounces) package cream cheese, softened

• 1/8 cup grated Parmesan cheese

• 1/8 teaspoon ground black pepper

• 1/8 teaspoon onion powder

• 1/8 teaspoon ground cayenne pepper

Directions:

• Preheat the oven to 350 degrees F. Spray a baking sheet with cooking spray. Clean mushrooms with a damp paper towel. Carefully break off stems. Chop stems extremely fine, discarding the tough end of stems.

23

• Heat oil in a large skillet over medium heat. Add garlic and chopped mushroom stems to the skillet. Fry until any moisture has disappeared, taking care not to burn the garlic. Set aside to cool.

• When garlic and mushroom mixture is no longer hot, stir in cream cheese, Parmesan cheese, black pepper, onion powder, and cayenne pepper. The mixture should be very thick. Using a little spoon, fill each mushroom cap with a generous amount of stuffing. Arrange the mushroom caps on the prepared cookie sheet.

• Bake for 20 minutes in the preheated oven, or until the mushrooms are piping hot and liquid starts to form under caps.

Nutrition:

Calories 150 | Total Fat 14.5g | Saturated Fat 8.6g | Cholesterol 42mg | Sodium 171mg | Total Carbohydrate 2g | Dietary Fiber 0.4g | Total Sugars 0.3g | Protein 3.6g | Calcium 37mg | Iron 1mg | Potassium 50mg | Phosphorus 10mg

Sautéed Mushrooms

Preparation Time: 10 minutes | Cooking Time: 15 minutes | Servings: 4

Ingredients:

- 3 tablespoons olive oil

- 3 tablespoons unsalted butter

- 1 pound button mushrooms, sliced

- 1 clove garlic, thinly sliced

- 1/8 teaspoon salt, or to taste

- Freshly ground black pepper to taste

Directions:

- Heat olive oil and unsalted butter in a large saucepan over medium heat. Cook and stir mushrooms, garlic, salt, and black pepper in the hot oil and butter until mushrooms are lightly browned, about 5 minutes. Reduce heat to low and simmer until mushrooms are tender, 5 to 8 more minutes.

Nutrition:

Calories 171 | Total Fat 19.2g | Saturated Fat 7g | Cholesterol 23mg | Sodium 62mg | Total Carbohydrate 0.9g | Dietary Fiber 0.2g | Total Sugars 0.3g | Protein 0.7g | Calcium 4mg | Iron 1mg | Potassium 62mg | Phosphorus 50 mg

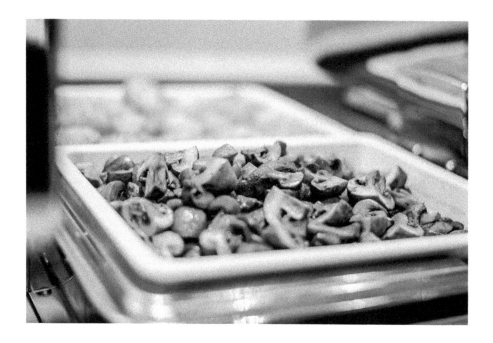

Mushroom Rice

Preparation Time: 05 minutes | Cooking Time: 25 minutes | Servings: 4

Ingredients:

- 2 teaspoons olive oil

- 6 mushrooms, coarsely chopped

- 1 clove garlic, minced

- 1 green onion, finely chopped

- 1 cup uncooked white rice

- 1/2 teaspoon chopped fresh parsley

- Salt and pepper to taste

- 1-1/2 cups water

Directions:

- Heat olive oil in a saucepan over medium heat. Cook mushrooms, garlic, and green onion until mushrooms are cooked and liquid has evaporated. Stir in water and rice. Season with parsley, salt, and pepper. Reduce heat, cover, and simmer for 20 minutes.

Nutrition:

Calories 197 | Total Fat 2.7g | Saturated Fat 0.4g | Cholesterol 0mg | Sodium 5mg | Total Carbohydrate 38.4g | Dietary Fiber 1g | Total Sugars 0.6g | Protein 4.3g | Calcium 17mg | Iron 3mg | Potassium 154mg | Phosphorus 110 mg

Roasted Asparagus and Mushrooms

Preparation Time: 10 minutes | Cooking Time: 15 minutes | Servings: 4

Ingredients:

• 1 bunch fresh asparagus, trimmed

• 1/2 pound fresh mushrooms, quartered

• 2 sprigs fresh rosemary, minced

• 2 teaspoons olive oil

• Freshly ground black pepper to taste

Directions:

• Preheat the oven to 450 degrees F. Lightly spray a cookie sheet with vegetable cooking spray.

• Place the asparagus and mushrooms in a bowl. Drizzle with the olive oil, then season with rosemary and pepper; toss well. Lay the asparagus and mushrooms out on the prepared pan in an even layer. Roast in the preheated oven until the asparagus is tender, about 15 minutes.

Nutrition:

Calories 31 | Total Fat 2.5g | Saturated Fat 0.4g | Cholesterol 0mg | Sodium 1mg | Total Carbohydrate 2g | Dietary Fiber 1.1g | Total Sugars 0.8g | Protein 1g | Calcium 16mg | Iron 1mg | Potassium 102mg | Phosphorus 70mg

Buckwheat Bake

Preparation Time: 10 minutes | Cooking Time: 1hr.15 minutes |
Servings: 4

Ingredients:

• 1/4 cup olive oil

• 1 medium onion, diced

• 1 cup uncooked buckwheat

• 2 green onions, thinly sliced

• 1/2 cup sliced fresh mushrooms

• 1/2 cup chopped fresh parsley

• 1/8 teaspoon salt

• 1/8 teaspoon pepper

• 2 water

Directions:

• Preheat the oven to 350 degrees F.

• Melt olive oil in a skillet over medium-high heat. Stir in onion, buckwheat. Cook and stir until buckwheat is lightly browned. Mix in green onions, mushrooms, and parsley. Season with salt and pepper. Transfer the mixture to a 2-quart casserole dish, and stir in the water.

• Bake 1 hour and 15 minutes in the preheated oven, or until liquid has been absorbed and

buckwheat is tender.

Nutrition:

Calories 181 | Total Fat 9.5g | Saturated Fat 1.4g | Cholesterol 0mg | Sodium 102mg | Total Carbohydrate 22.9g | Dietary Fiber 3.6g | Total Sugars 1g | Protein 4.4g | Calcium 20mg | Iron 1mg | Potassium 218mg | Phosphorus 170 mg

Stir-Fry Vegetables

Preparation Time: 10 minutes | Cooking Time: 20 minutes | Servings: 4

Ingredients:

- 2 cups green pepper

- 2 cups red pepper

- 1 cup fresh sliced mushrooms

- 1 cup celery

- ¼ cup onion

- 1 garlic clove

- ½ teaspoon honey

- ½ teaspoon dried oregano

- 1/8 teaspoon salt

- 1/8 teaspoon pepper

- 1 tablespoon olive oil

Directions:

• Cut green and red peppers. Slice celery and chop onion. Crush garlic.

• In a large skillet, heat oil. Add green pepper, red pepper, mushrooms, celery, onion, garlic, honey, oregano, salt, and pepper.

• Stir-fry over medium-high heat until peppers are crisp-tender.

• Serve hot.

Nutrition:

Calories 36 | Total Fat 1.6g | Saturated Fat 0.2g | Cholesterol 0mg | Sodium 69mg | Total Carbohydrate 5.4g | Dietary Fiber 1.2g | Total Sugars 2.6g | Protein 0.9g | Calcium 13mg | Iron 1mg | Potassium 162mg | Phosphorus 120mg

Roasted Apples and Cabbage

Preparation Time: 15 minutes | Cooking Time: 20 minutes | Servings: 4

Ingredients:

- 1 cup chopped cabbage

- 2 apples - peeled, cored, and cut into 3/4-inch chunks

- 2 tablespoons olive oil, or as needed

- Salt and ground black pepper to taste

- 1 pinch garlic powder to taste

- Zest from 1 lemon

- Juice from 1 lemon

Directions:

- Preheat the oven to 425 degrees F.

- Arrange cabbage in a single layer on a rimmed baking sheet; sprinkle apple pieces evenly around the baking sheet. Drizzle the cabbage, apples with olive oil; sprinkle with salt, black pepper, and garlic powder. Toss the mixture gently to coat.

• Roast in the preheated oven until the cabbage is hot and fragrant, about 20 minutes. Sprinkle with lemon zest, and squeeze juice from zested lemon over the cabbage to serve.

Nutrition:

Calories 127 | Total Fat 7.3g | Saturated Fat 1g | Cholesterol 0mg | Sodium 4mg | Total Carbohydrate 17.8g | Dietary Fiber 3.6g | Total Sugars 12.5g | Protein 0.7g | Calcium 11mg | Iron 1mg | Potassium 170mg | Phosphorus 80mg

Cabbage Bake

Preparation Time: 15 minutes | Cooking Time: 30 minutes | Servings: 4

Ingredients:

- 1 cup of water

- 1 cup cabbage

- ½ tablespoon olive oil

- 1 egg, beaten

- ½ cup shredded Cheddar cheese

- ½ cup graham crackers

Directions:

- Preheat the oven to 350 degrees F.

- Bring water to boil in a medium saucepan. Place chopped cabbage in the water, and return to boil. Reduce heat, and simmer 2 minutes, until tender; drain.

- In a medium bowl, mix cabbage with oil, egg, Cheddar cheese, and 1/3 cup graham crackers.

Transfer to a medium baking dish and top with remaining graham crackers.

• Cover, and bake for 25 minutes in the preheated oven, until bubbly. Uncover, and continue baking 5 minutes, until lightly browned.

Nutrition:

Calories 91 | Total Fat 5.7g | Saturated Fat 2.5g | Cholesterol 37mg | Sodium 114mg | Total Carbohydrate 6.2g | Dietary Fiber 0.5g | Total Sugars 2.7g | Protein 3.9g | Calcium 79mg | Iron 1mg | Potassium 49mg | Phosphorus 20mg

Zippy Zucchini

Preparation Time: 10 minutes | | Cooking Time: 15 minutes | Servings: 4

Ingredients:

- 2 cups zucchini

- ½ medium onion

- 2 large eggs

- ¼ cup shredded cheddar cheese

- 1/8 teaspoon salt

- 1/8 teaspoon black pepper

Directions:

- Cut zucchini into chunks. Thinly slice the onion.

- Place zucchini and onion in a 10‖ x 6‖ x 2‖ dish. Cover with plastic wrap, turning one edge back slightly to vent. Microwave on high for 7 minutes. Drain liquid.

- In a large bowl, mix beaten eggs, cheese, salt, and pepper. Add zucchini and onions, stirring well.

• Grease dish in which vegetables were microwaved.

• Pour mixture into a dish and cover with a paper towel. Microwave on medium-high for 4 minutes. Remove the paper towel and stir.

• Continue to microwave uncovered for 4 to 6 minutes until the center is set.

Nutrition:

Calories 80 | Total Fat 5g | Saturated Fat 2.3g | Cholesterol 100mg | Sodium 159mg | Total Carbohydrate 3.7g | Dietary Fiber 1g | Total Sugars 1.9g | Protein 5.8g | Calcium 77mg | Iron 1mg | Potassium 224mg | Phosphorus 124 mg

Barley with Beans

Preparation Time: 10 minutes | | Cooking Time: 20 minutes | Servings: 4

Ingredients:

- 1 tablespoon olive oil

- 1 cup uncooked barley

- 2 cups of water

- 1/4 cup chopped onion

- 1 clove garlic, minced

- 1 teaspoon chopped fresh basil

- 1/2 teaspoon black pepper

- 3/4 cup green beans

- 1/2 cup grated parmesan cheese, divided

- 2 tablespoons chopped fresh parsley

Directions:

• Heat the oil in a saucepan over medium heat. Stir in the barley, and cook for 2 minutes until toasted. Pour in the water, onion, garlic, basil, and black pepper. Cover, and let come to a boil. Once boiling, stir in the green beans. Recover, reduce heat to medium-low, and continue simmering until the barley is tender and has absorbed the water, 15 to 20 minutes.

• Stir in half of the parmesan cheese and the parsley until evenly mixed. Scoop the barley into a serving dish, and sprinkle with the remaining parmesan cheese to serve.

Nutrition:

Calories 155 | Total Fat 3.6g | Saturated Fat 0.8g | Cholesterol 2mg | Sodium 43mg | Total Carbohydrate 26.3g | Dietary Fiber 6.6g | Total Sugars 1.4g | Protein 5.8g | Calcium 43mg | Iron 2mg | Potassium 180mg | Phosphorus 120 mg

Zucchini Stir-Fry

Preparation Time: 10 minutes | Cooking Time: 05 minutes | Servings: 4

Ingredients:

- 1 tablespoon olive oil

- 1 teaspoon cumin

- 2 cups zucchini

- 1/2 cup red onion

- 1 teaspoon black pepper

- 1 tablespoon lemon juice

- 1/4 cup fresh parsley

Directions:

- Peel and slice zucchini and onion. Chop parsley.

- Heat olive oil in a non-stick skillet over medium heat.

- Sauté cumin to brown.

- Add zucchini and onion and sprinkle with black pepper. Stir a few times to mix.

• Cover and cook for approximately 5 minutes to medium tenderness, stirring a few times. • Add lemon juice and chopped parsley. Mix, cook another minute, and serve.

Nutrition:

Calories 51 | Total Fat 3.8g | Saturated Fat 0.6g | Cholesterol 0mg | Sodium 11mg | Total Carbohydrate 4.3g | Dietary Fiber 1.3g | Total Sugars 1.8g | Protein 1.2g | Calcium 25mg | Iron 1mg | Potassium 225mg | Phosphorus 108 mg

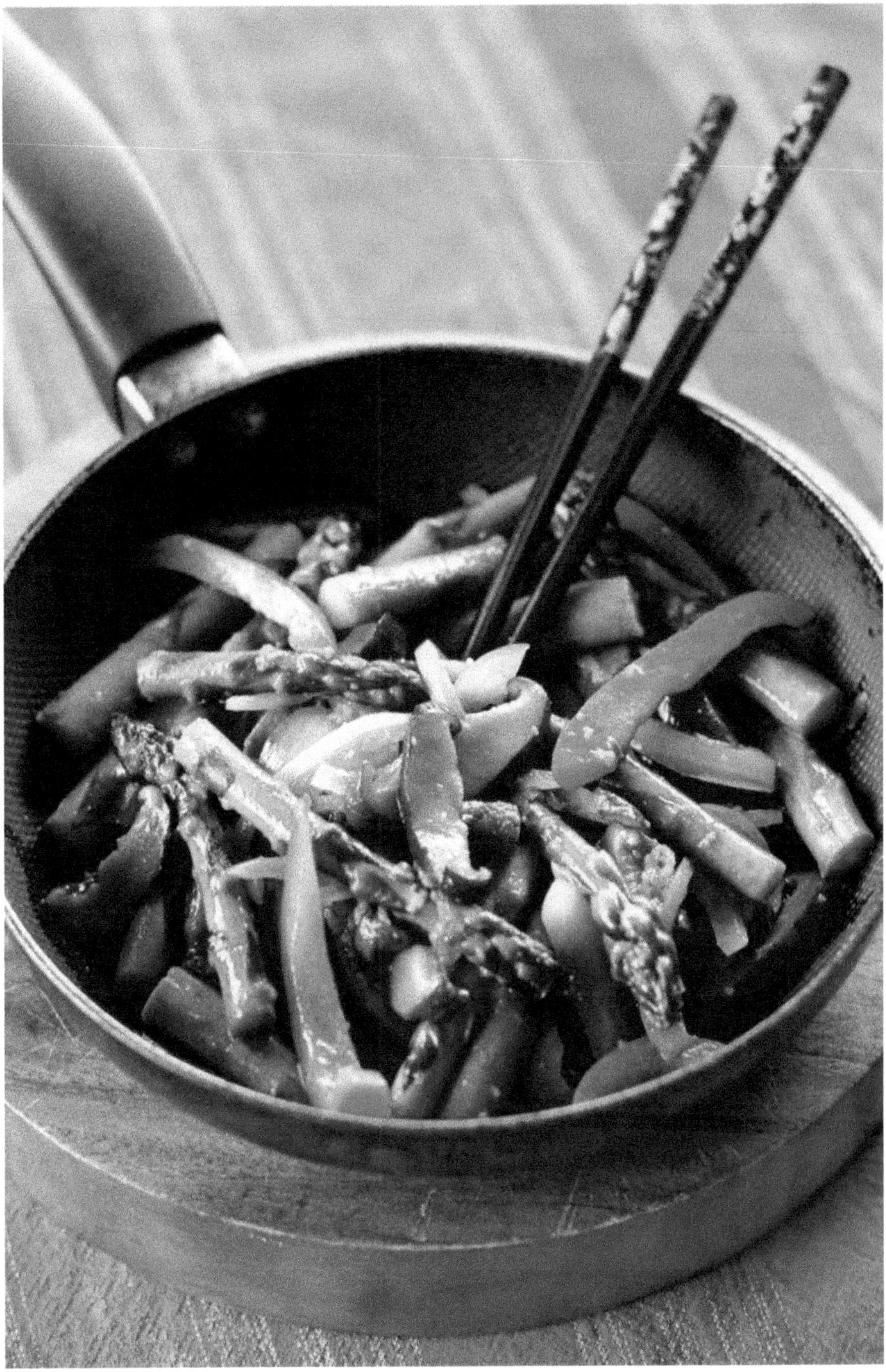

Couscous Primavera

Preparation Time: 15 minutes | Cooking Time: 20 minutes | Servings: 4

Ingredients:

- 1 cup dry couscous

- ½ cup broccoli

- 1/2 cup chopped green onions

- 2 tablespoons olive oil

- 1/2 teaspoon ground cumin

- 1 pinch ground black pepper

- 2 cups of water

- 1 bunch asparagus, trimmed and cut into 1/4-inch pieces

- 1 cup shelled fresh or thawed frozen beans

- 2 tablespoons chopped fresh basil

- Salt and freshly ground black pepper to taste

Directions:

• Combine couscous, green onion, broccoli, olive oil, cumin, and black pepper in a large bowl; stir until the olive oil is completely incorporated.

• Bring water, asparagus, and beans to a boil in a saucepan over high heat.

• Pour water, asparagus, and peas over couscous mixture; shake the bowl to settle couscous into liquid. Cover and let stand for 10 minutes. Fluff with a fork, then stir in basil and season with salt and pepper to taste.

Nutrition:

Calories 174 | Total Fat 5g | Saturated Fat 0.7g | Cholesterol 0mg | Sodium 57mg | Total Carbohydrate 26.9g | Dietary Fiber 3.2g | Total Sugars 1.6g | Protein 5.6g | Calcium 24mg | Iron 1mg | Potassium 124mg | Phosphorus 108 mg

Lemon Pepper Beans

Preparation Time: 01 minutes | Cooking Time: 05 minutes | Servings: 4

Ingredients:

- 1 cup frozen green beans, thawed

- 1 tablespoon water

- 2 tablespoons olive oil

- 1 pinch lemon pepper

- 1 pinch dried rosemary

Directions:

• Place the beans and water into a microwave-safe bowl. Cover loosely, and microwave for 3 to 4 minutes, or until beans are tender. Stir in oil, and sprinkle with lemon pepper and rosemary. Serve warm.

Nutrition:

Calories 90 | Total Fat 7.2g | Saturated Fat 1g | Cholesterol 0mg | Sodium 2mg | Total Carbohydrate 5.3g | Dietary Fiber 1.9g | Total Sugars 2.1g | Protein 2g | Calcium 10mg | Iron 1mg | Potassium 89mg | Phosphorus 45 mg

Sweet Bean and Noodles

Preparation Time: 15 minutes | Cooking Time: 15 minutes | Servings: 4

Ingredients:

• 12 ounces egg noodle

• 1 cup green beans

• 1 onion, chopped

• 1/2 cup mayonnaise

• 1 dash black pepper

Directions:

• In a large pot of boiling water, cook noodles until al dente, rinse under cold water and drain.

• In a mixing bowl, combine the noodle, green beans, onions, mayonnaise, and a dash of black pepper. Mix well and chill before serving.

Nutrition:

Calories 265 | Total Fat 11.7g | Saturated Fat 1.8g | Cholesterol 31mg | Sodium 106mg | Total Carbohydrate 35g | Dietary Fiber 3.4g | Total Sugars 5.4g | Protein 6.2g | Calcium 29mg | Iron 1mg | Potassium 81mg | Phosphorus 25 mg

Bean Rice

Preparation Time: 15 minutes | Cooking Time: 20 minutes | Servings: 4

Ingredients:

- 1 cup white rice
- 1 tablespoon olive oil
- 2 whole cloves
- 1 (2-inch) piece of cinnamon stick
- 1 bell pepper, chopped
- 1 teaspoon minced fresh ginger root
- ¼ cup green beans
- ¼ teaspoon honey
- 2 cups of water

Directions:

- Wash and drain the rice.

• Heat a saucepan over medium heat. Add olive oil and let heat it. Stir in cloves, cinnamon, bell pepper, and ginger. Sauté briefly. Mix in rice and stir to coat it evenly. Stir in beans, honey. Pour in water and bring the water to a boil.

• Reduce heat to simmer and let rice cook covered for 15 to 20 minutes; or until rice is tender.

Nutrition:

Calories 224 | Total Fat 4.2g | Saturated Fat 0.7g | Cholesterol 0mg | Sodium 10mg | Total Carbohydrate 42.5g | Dietary Fiber 2.4g | Total Sugars 2.5g | Protein 4.2g | Calcium 40mg | Iron 2mg | Potassium 151mg | Phosphorus 125 mg

Fried Cabbage

Preparation Time: 05 minutes | Cooking Time: 45 minutes | Servings: 4

Ingredients:

• 2 teaspoons olive oil

• 1 cup of water

• 1 head cabbage, cored and coarsely chopped

• 1 pinch salt and pepper to taste

Directions:

• Bring the oil and water to a boil in a large skillet. Reduce heat to low and add the cabbage. Cover and cook over low heat to steam the cabbage for about 45 minutes, stirring frequently, or until the cabbage is tender and sweet. Season with salt and pepper and serve.

Nutrition:

Calories 43 | Total Fat 1.7g | Saturated Fat 0.3g | Cholesterol 0mg | Sodium 21mg | Total Carbohydrate 6.9g | Dietary Fiber 3g

| Total Sugars 3.8g | Protein 1.5g | Calcium 48mg | Iron 1mg | Potassium 202mg | Phosphorus 100 mg

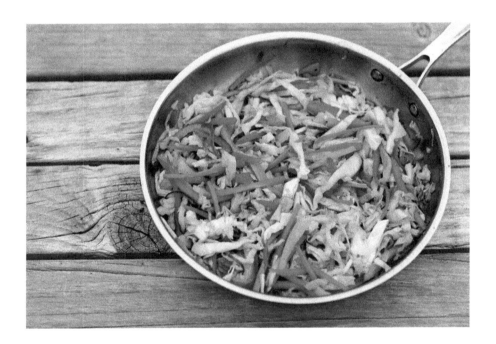

Roasted Cabbage

Preparation Time: 10 minutes | Cooking Time: 30 minutes | Servings: 4

Ingredients:

- 2 tablespoons butter

- 1/2 head green cabbage, cut into 4 wedges

- 1 pinch garlic powder, or to taste

- 1 pinch red pepper flakes, or to taste

- Salt and ground black pepper to taste

- 2 lemons, halved

Directions:

- Preheat the oven to 450 degrees F.

- Brush both sides of each cabbage wedge with melted butter. Sprinkle garlic powder, red pepper flakes, salt, and pepper over each wedge. Arrange wedges on a baking sheet.

• Roast in the preheated oven for 15 minutes; flip cabbage and continue roasting until browned and charred in some areas, about 15 minutes more. Squeeze lemon over each wedge.

Nutrition:

Calories 89 | Total Fat 6g | Saturated Fat 3.7g | Cholesterol 15mg | Sodium 58mg | Total Carbohydrate 9.4g | Dietary Fiber 3.3g | Total Sugars 3.6g | Protein 1.8g | Calcium 48mg | Iron 1mg | Potassium 195mg | Phosphorus 90 mg

Okra Buckwheat

Preparation Time: 10 minutes | Cooking Time: 30 minutes | Servings: 4

Ingredients:

- 1 large onion, chopped

- 3 cups sliced fresh okra

- 1 cup of water

- ½ teaspoon olive oil

- 1 cup uncooked buckwheat

Directions:

• In the skillet, heat olive oil and sauté onion over medium-high heat until tender, about 3 minutes. Sliced okra, and water. Reduce heat and simmer until okra is tender and falling apart, about 15 minutes. Stir in buckwheat and water. Cover, and simmer for 20 minutes, or until fluffy.

Nutrition:

Calories 127 | Total Fat 1.1g | Saturated Fat 0.2g | Cholesterol 0mg | Sodium 6mg | Total Carbohydrate 26.3g | Dietary Fiber 5g | Total Sugars 1.8g | Protein 5g | Calcium 53mg | Iron 1mg | Potassium 317mg | Phosphorus 190 mg

Black Beans, Corn, and Yellow Rice

Preparation Time: 10 minutes | Cooking Time: 25 minutes | Servings: 8

Ingredients:

• 8 ounces yellow rice mix

• 15.25 ounces cooked kernel corn

• 1 1/4 cups water

• 15 ounces cooked black beans

• 1 teaspoon ground cumin

• 2 teaspoons lime juice

• 2 tablespoons olive oil

Directions:

• Place a saucepan over high heat, add oil, water, and rice, bring the mixture to a bowl, and then switch heat to medium-low level.

• Simmer for 25 minutes until rice is tender and all the liquid has been absorbed and then transfer the rice to a large bowl.

• Add remaining ingredients into the rice, stir until mixed and serve straight away.

Nutrition:

Calories: 100 Cal | Fat: 4.4 g | Carbs: 15.1 g | Protein: 2 g | Fiber: 1.4 g

Okra Curry

Preparation Time: 05 minutes | Cooking Time: 10 minutes | Servings: 4

Ingredients:

- 1 pound okra, ends trimmed, cut into 1/4-inch rounds

- 1 tablespoon olive oil

- 1/2 teaspoon curry powder

- 1/2 teaspoon all-purpose flour

- 1/2 teaspoon black pepper

Directions:

- Microwave the okra on High for 3 minutes.

- Heat olive oil in a large skillet over medium heat. Gently mix in the curry powder, all-purpose flour, and black pepper; cook 2 minutes more. Serve immediately.

Nutrition:

Calories 45 | Total Fat 3.7g | Saturated Fat 0.5g | Cholesterol 0mg | Sodium 3mg | Total Carbohydrate 2.7g | Dietary Fiber 1g | Total Sugars 0.4g | Protein 0.7g | Calcium 28mg | Iron 1mg | Potassium 92mg | Phosphorus 60 mg

Frying Pan Okra

Preparation Time: 05 minutes | Cooking Time: 10 minutes | Servings: 4

Ingredients:

• 1 tablespoon olive oil

• 2 onions, sliced

• ½ pound fresh okra, sliced into 1/8-inch pieces

• ½ teaspoon ground turmeric

Directions:

• Heat olive oil in a medium saucepan over medium heat and sauté onion until translucent. Stir in okra and turmeric. Reduce heat to low and cook for 15 minutes, or until tender.

Nutrition:

Calories 32 | Total Fat 1.8g | Saturated Fat 0.3g | Cholesterol 0mg | Sodium 2mg | Total Carbohydrate 3.6g | Dietary Fiber 1g | Total Sugars 1.4g | Protein 0.6g | Calcium 17mg | Iron 0mg | Potassium 81mg | Phosphorus 50 mg

Lemony Grilled Okra

Preparation Time: 10min | Cooking Time: 10 minutes | Servings: 4

Ingredients:

- 1 pound okra, stems trimmed

- 1 tablespoon olive oil, or more as needed

- 1 pinch paprika, or to taste

- 1 pinch garlic powder, or to taste

- Salt and freshly ground black pepper to taste

- 1 pinch cayenne pepper

- 1 lemon, juiced

- 1/4 teaspoon chopped fresh dill, or to taste

- 1/4 teaspoon chopped fresh basil, or to taste

Directions:

- Preheat an outdoor grill for high heat and lightly oil the grate.

• Toss okra with olive oil, paprika, garlic powder, salt, pepper, and cayenne pepper in a bowl.

• Grill okra on the preheated grill until 1 side is bright green with visible grill marks, about 5 minutes. Turn okra, cover grill, and cook until tender, about 5 minutes.

• Transfer okra to a serving bowl; sprinkle with lemon juice, dill weed, and basil.

Nutrition:

Calories 45 | Total Fat 3.6g | Saturated Fat 0.5g | Cholesterol 0mg | Sodium 2mg | Total Carbohydrate 3.4g | Dietary Fiber 1.3g | Total Sugars 0.8g | Protein 0.7g | Calcium 26mg | Iron 0mg | Potassium 101mg | Phosphorus 90 mg

Stuffed Okra

Preparation Time: 15min | Cooking Time: 05 minutes | Servings: 4

Ingredients:

- 1 teaspoon ground ginger

- 1 teaspoon ground cumin

- 1 teaspoon ground turmeric

- 1/2 teaspoon chili powder (optional)

- 1/8 teaspoon salt

- 1/2 teaspoon butter

- 1 pound large okra

- 1/4 cup all-purpose flour

- Olive oil for frying

Directions:

• Combine ginger, cumin, turmeric, chili powder, salt, and 1/2 teaspoon butter in a bowl; set aside for flavors to blend for 2 hours.

• Heat olive oil in a deep-fryer or large saucepan to 350 degrees F.

• Trim okra and make a slit lengthwise down the side of each okra, creating a pocket. Fill each pocket with the spice mixture.

• Place all-purpose flour in a resealable plastic bag; add filled okra and shake to coat.

• Fry okra in the hot oil until golden brown, 5 to 8 minutes. Transfer fried okra using a slotted spoon to a paper towel-lined plate.

Nutrition:

Calories 43 | Total Fat 0.5g | Saturated Fat 0.2g | Cholesterol 1mg | Sodium 43mg | Total Carbohydrate 8g | Dietary Fiber 2.1g | Total Sugars 1.1g | Protein 1.6g | Calcium 51mg | Iron 1mg | Potassium 194mg | Phosphorus 80 mg

Mashed Turnip

Preparation Time: 10 minutes | Cooking Time: 50 minutes | Servings: 4

Ingredients:

- 1 large turnip, peeled and cubed

- 1 cup cauliflower

- 1/4 cup soy milk

- 1 tablespoon olive oil

- 1 teaspoon honey

- 1/8 teaspoon salt

- 1/4 teaspoon pepper

Directions:

- Preheat the oven to 375 degrees F.

- Place turnip and cauliflower in a large pot with enough water to cover, and bring to a boil.

- Cook for 25 to 30 minutes, until tender. Remove from heat, and drain.

- Mix soy milk, ¼ tablespoon olive oil, and honey with the turnip and cauliflower. Season with salt and pepper. Mash until slightly lumpy.

- Transfer turnip mixture to a small baking dish. Dot with remaining olive oil. Cover loosely, and bake 15 minutes in the preheated oven. Remove cover, and continue baking for about 8 minutes, until lightly browned.

Nutrition:

Calories 42 | Total Fat 2.6g | Saturated Fat 0.4g | Cholesterol 0mg | Sodium 321mg | Total Carbohydrate 4.5g | Dietary Fiber 1.1g | Total Sugars 2.9g | Protein 0.9g | Calcium 16mg | Iron 0mg | Potassium 123mg | Phosphorus 70 mg

Sautéed Zucchini and Leeks

Preparation Time: 15 minutes | Cooking Time: 20 minutes | Servings: 4

Ingredients:

- 2 leeks, finely chopped

- 2 zucchini, finely chopped

- 1/3 cup water

- 2 tablespoons olive oil

- 1 tablespoon honey

- 1/2 teaspoon dried basil

- Pinch of salt

- 1/8 teaspoon ground black pepper

Directions:

• Combine leeks, zucchinis, water, olive oil, honey, basil, salt, and pepper in a skillet; bring to a boil. Reduce heat and simmer until liquid evaporates for about 15 minutes. Cook and stir mixture until leeks and carrots are lightly browned, 2 to 3 minutes.

Nutrition:

Calories 79 | Total Fat 4.9g | Saturated Fat 0.7g | Cholesterol 0mg | Sodium 40mg | Total Carbohydrate 9.3g, | Dietary Fiber 1.3g | Total Sugars 5.2g, | Protein 1.3g | Calcium 28mg | Iron 1mg | Potassium 227mg | Phosphorus 180 mg

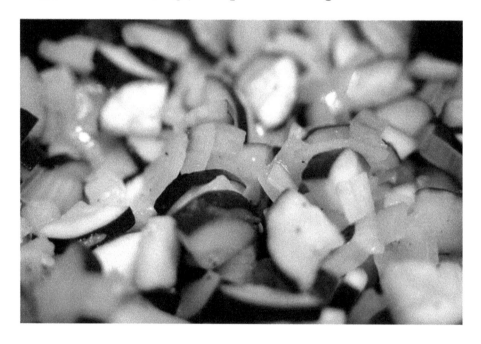

Black Beans and Rice

Preparation Time: 10 minutes | Cooking Time: 30 minutes | Servings: 4

Ingredients:

- 3/4 cup white rice

- 1 medium white onion, peeled, chopped

- 3 1/2 cups cooked black beans

- 1 teaspoon minced garlic

- 1/4 teaspoon cayenne pepper

- 1 teaspoon ground cumin

- 1 teaspoon olive oil

- 1 1/2 cups vegetable broth

Directions:

• Take a large pot over medium-high heat, add oil and when hot, add onion and garlic and cook for 4 minutes until saute.

• Then stir in rice, cook for 2 minutes, pour in the broth, bring it to a boil, switch heat to the low level and cook for 20 minutes until tender.

• Stir in remaining ingredients, cook for 2 minutes, and then serve straight away.

Nutrition:

Calories: 140 Cal | Fat: 0.9 g | Carbs: 27.1 g | Protein: 6.3 g | Fiber: 6.2 g

Brown Rice Pilaf

Preparation Time: 5 minutes | Cooking Time: 25 minutes | Servings: 4

Ingredients:

- 1 cup cooked chickpeas

- 3/4 cup brown rice, cooked

- 1/4 cup chopped cashews

- 2 cups sliced mushrooms

- 2 carrots, sliced

- ½ teaspoon minced garlic

- 1 1/2 cups chopped white onion

- 3 tablespoons vegan butter

- ½ teaspoon salt

- ¼ teaspoon ground black pepper

- 1/4 cup chopped parsley

Directions:

• Take a large skillet pan, place it over medium heat, add butter and when it melts, add onions and cook them for 5 minutes until softened.

• Then add carrots and garlic, cook for 5 minutes, add mushrooms, cook for 10 minutes until browned, add chickpeas and cook for another minute.

• When done, remove the pan from heat, add nuts, parsley, salt, and black pepper, toss until mixed, and garnish with parsley.

• Serve straight away.

Nutrition:

Calories: 409 Cal | Fat: 17.1 g | Carbs: 54 g | Protein: 12.5 g | Fiber: 6.7 g

Barley and Mushrooms with Beans

Preparation Time: 5 minutes | Cooking Time: 15 minutes | Servings: 6

Ingredients:

- 1/2 cup uncooked barley

- 15.5 ounces white beans

- 1/2 cup chopped celery

- 3 cups sliced mushrooms

- 1 cup chopped white onion

- 1 teaspoon minced garlic

- 1 teaspoon olive oil

- 3 cups vegetable broth

Directions:

• Take a saucepan, place it over medium heat, add oil and when hot, add vegetables and cook for 5 minutes until tender.

• Pour in broth, stir in barley, bring the mixture to boil, and then simmer for 50 minutes until tender.

• When done, add beans into the barley mixture, stir until mixed and continue cooking for 5 minutes until hot.

• Serve straight away.

Nutrition:

Calories: 202 Cal | Fat: 2.1 g | Carbs: 39 g | Protein: 9.1 g | Fiber: 8.8 g

Vegan Curried Rice

Preparation Time: 5 minutes | Cooking Time: 25 minutes | Servings: 4

Ingredients:

- 1 cup white rice

- 1 tablespoon minced garlic

- 1 tablespoon ground curry powder

- 1/3 teaspoon ground black pepper

- 1 tablespoon red chili powder

- 1 tablespoon ground cumin

- 2 tablespoons olive oil

- 1 tablespoon soy sauce

- 1 cup vegetable broth

Directions:

• Take a saucepan, place it over low heat, add oil and when hot, add garlic and cook for 3 minutes.

• Then stir in all spices, cook for 1 minute until fragrant, pour in the broth, and switch heat to a high level.

• Stir in soy sauce, bring the mixture to boil, add rice, stir until mixed, then switch heat to the low level and simmer for 20 minutes until rice is tender and all the liquid has absorbed.

• Serve straight away.

Nutrition:

Calories: 262 Cal | Fat: 8 g | Carbs: 43 g | Protein: 5 g | Fiber: 2 g

Lentils and Rice with Fried Onions

Preparation Time: 5 minutes | Cooking Time: 7 minutes | Servings: 4

Ingredients:

- 3/4 cup long-grain white rice, cooked

- 1 large white onion, peeled, sliced

- 1 1/3 cups green lentils, cooked

- ½ teaspoon salt

- 1/4 cup vegan sour cream

- ¼ teaspoon ground black pepper

- 6 tablespoons olive oil

Directions:

• Take a large skillet pan, place it over medium heat, add oil, and when hot, add onions, and cook for 10 minutes until browned, set aside until required.

• Take a saucepan, place it over medium heat, grease it with oil, add lentils and beans and cook for 3 minutes until warmed.

• Season with salt and black pepper, cook for 2 minutes, then stir in half of the browned onions, and top with cream and remaining onions.

• Serve straight away.

Nutrition:

Calories: 535 Cal | Fat: 22.1 g | Carbs: 69 g | Protein: 17.3 g | Fiber: 10.6 g

Asparagus Rice Pilaf

Preparation Time: 10 minutes | Cooking Time: 35 minutes | Servings: 4

Ingredients:

- 1 1/4 cups rice

- 1/2 pound asparagus, diced, boiled

- 2 ounces spaghetti, whole-grain, broken

- 1/4 cup minced white onion

- 1/2 teaspoon minced garlic

- 1/2 cup cashew halves

- ¼ teaspoon ground black pepper

- ½ teaspoon salt

- 1/4 cup vegan butter

- 2 1/4 cups vegetable broth

Directions:

• Take a saucepan, place it over medium-low heat, add butter and when it melts, stir in spaghetti and cook for 3 minutes until golden brown.

• Add onion and garlic, cook for 2 minutes until tender, then stir in rice, cook for 5 minutes, pour in the broth, season with salt and black pepper, and bring it to a boil.

• Switch heat to medium level, cook for 20 minutes, then add cashews and asparagus, and stir until combined.

• Serve straight away.

Nutrition:

Calories: 249 Cal | Fat: 10 g | Carbs: 35.1 g | Protein: 5.3 g | Fiber: 1.8 g

Mexican Stuffed Peppers

Preparation Time: 10 minutes | Cooking Time: 40 minutes | Servings: 4

Ingredients:

- 2 cups cooked rice

- 1/2 cup chopped onion

- 15 ounces cooked black beans

- 4 large green bell peppers, destemmed, cored

- 1 tablespoon olive oil

- 1 tablespoon salt

- 14.5 ounce diced tomatoes

- 1/2 teaspoon ground cumin

- 1 teaspoon garlic salt

- 1 teaspoon red chili powder

- 1/2 teaspoon salt

- 2 cups shredded vegan Mexican cheese blend

Directions:

• Boil the bell peppers in salty water for 5 minutes until softened and then set aside until required.

• Heat oil over medium heat in a skillet pan, then add onion and cook for 10 minutes until softened.

• Transfer the onion mixture in a bowl, add remaining ingredients, reserving ½ cup cheese blended, stir until mixed, and then fill this mixture into the boiled peppers.

• Arrange the peppers in the square baking dish, sprinkle them with remaining cheese and bake for 30 minutes at 350 degrees F.

• Serve straight away.

Nutrition:

Calories: 509 Cal | Fat: 22.8 g | Carbs: 55.5 g | Protein: 24 g | Fiber: 12 g

Quinoa and Black Bean Chili

Preparation Time: 10 minutes | Cooking Time: 32 minutes | Servings: 10

Ingredients:

- 1 cup quinoa, cooked

- 38 ounces cooked black beans

- 1 medium white onion, peeled, chopped

- 1 cup of frozen corn

- 1 green bell pepper, deseeded, chopped

- 1 zucchini, chopped

- 1 tablespoon minced chipotle peppers in adobo sauce

- 1 red bell pepper, deseeded, chopped

- 1 jalapeno pepper, deseeded, minced

- 28 ounces crushed tomatoes

- 2 teaspoons minced garlic

- 1/3 teaspoon ground black pepper

- ¾ teaspoon salt

- 1 teaspoon dried oregano

- 1 tablespoon red chili powder

- 1 tablespoon ground cumin

- 1 tablespoon olive oil

- 1/4 cup chopped cilantro

Directions:

• Take a large pot, place it over medium heat, add oil, and when hot, add onion and cook for 5 minutes.

• Then stir in garlic, cumin, and chili powder, cook for 1 minute, add remaining ingredients except for corn and quinoa, stir well and simmer for 20 minutes at medium-low heat until cooked.

• Then stir in corn and quinoa, cook for 5 minutes until hot and then top with cilantro.

• Serve straight away.

Nutrition:

Calories: 233 Cal | Fat: 3.5 g | Carbs: 42 g | Protein: 11.5 g | Fiber: 11.8 g

Mushroom Risotto

Preparation Time: 10 minutes | Cooking Time: 35 minutes | Servings: 4

Ingredients:

- 1 cup of rice

- 3 small white onions, peeled, chopped

- 1 teaspoon minced celery

- 1 ½ cups sliced mushrooms

- ½ teaspoon minced garlic

- 1 teaspoon minced parsley

- ½ teaspoon salt

- ¼ teaspoon ground black pepper

- 1 tablespoon olive oil

- 1 teaspoon vegan butter

- ¼ cup vegan cashew cream

- 1 cup grated vegan Parmesan cheese

- 1 cup of coconut milk

- 5 cups vegetable stock

Directions:

• Take a large skillet pan, place it over medium-high heat, add oil, and when hot, add onion and garlic and cook for 5 minutes.

• Transfer to a plate, add celery and parsley into the pan, stir in salt and black pepper, and cook for 3 minutes.

• Then switch heat to medium-low level, stir in mushrooms, cook for 5 minutes, then pour in cream and milk, stir in rice until combined, and bring the mixture to simmer.

• Pour in vegetable stock, one cup at a time until it has absorbed, and, when done, stir in cheese and butter.

• Serve straight away.

Nutrition:

Calories: 439 Cal | Fat: 19.5 g | Carbs: 48.7 g | Protein: 17 g | Fiber: 2 g

Quinoa with Chickpeas and Tomatoes

Preparation Time: 10 minutes | Cooking Time: 0 minute | Servings: 6

Ingredients:

- 1 tomato, chopped

- 1 cup quinoa, cooked

- ½ teaspoon minced garlic

- ¼ teaspoon ground black pepper

- ½ teaspoon salt

- 1/2 teaspoon ground cumin

- 4 teaspoons olive oil

- 3 tablespoons lime juice

- 1/2 teaspoon chopped parsley

Directions:

• Take a large bowl, place all the ingredients in it, except for the parsley, and stir until mixed.

• Garnish with parsley and serve straight away.

Nutrition:

Calories: 185 | Cal Fat: 5.4 g | Carbs: 28.8 g | Protein: 6 g | Fiber: 4.5 g

Barley Bake

Preparation Time: 10 minutes | Cooking Time: 98 minutes | Servings: 6

Ingredients:

- 1 cup pearl barley

- 1 medium white onion, peeled, diced

- 2 green onions, sliced

- 1/2 cup sliced mushrooms

- 1/8 teaspoon ground black pepper

- 1/4 teaspoon salt

- 1/2 cup chopped parsley

- 1/2 cup pine nuts

- 1/4 cup vegan butter

- 29 ounces vegetable broth

Directions:

• Place a skillet pan over medium-high heat, add butter and when it melts, stir in onion and barley, add nuts and cook for 5 minutes until light brown.

• Add mushrooms, green onions, and parsley, sprinkle with salt and black pepper, cook for 1 minute and then transfer the mixture into a casserole dish.

• Pour in broth, stir until mixed and bake for 90 minutes until barley is tender and has absorbed all the liquid.

• Serve straight away.

Nutrition:

Calories: 280 Cal | Fat: 14.2 g | Carbs: 33.2 g | Protein: 7.4 g | Fiber: 7 g

Zucchini Risotto

Preparation Time: 10 minutes | Cooking Time: 30 minutes | Servings: 6

Ingredients:

- 2 cups Arborio rice

- 10 sun-dried tomatoes, chopped

- 1 medium white onion, peeled, chopped

- 1 tablespoon chopped basil leaves

- 1/2 medium zucchini, sliced

- 1 teaspoon dried thyme

- 1/3 teaspoon ground black pepper

- 1 tablespoon vegan butter

- 6 tablespoons grated vegan Parmesan cheese

- 7 cups vegetable broth, hot

Directions:

• Take a large pot, place it over medium heat, add butter and when it melts, add onion and cook for 2 minutes.

• Stir in rice, cook for another 2 minutes until toasted, and then stir in broth, 1 cup at a time until absorbed completely and creamy mixture comes together.

• Then stir in remaining ingredients until combined, taste to adjust seasoning, and serve.

Nutrition:

Calories: 363 Cal | Fat: 4.1 g | Carbs: 71.2 g | Protein: 9.1 g | Fiber: 3.1 g

Lemony Quinoa

Preparation Time: 10 minutes | Cooking Time: 0 minute | Servings: 6

Ingredients:

- 1 cup quinoa, cooked

- 1/4 of medium red onion, peeled, chopped

- 1 bunch of parsley, chopped

- 2 stalks of celery, chopped

- ¼ teaspoon of sea salt

- 1/4 teaspoon cayenne pepper

- 1/2 teaspoon ground cumin

- 1/4 cup lemon juice

- 1/4 cup pine nuts, toasted

- Take a large bowl, place all the ingredients in it, and stir until combined.

- Serve straight away.

Nutrition:

Calories: 147 Cal | Fat: 4.8 g | Carbs: 21.4 g | Protein: 6 g | Fiber: 3 g

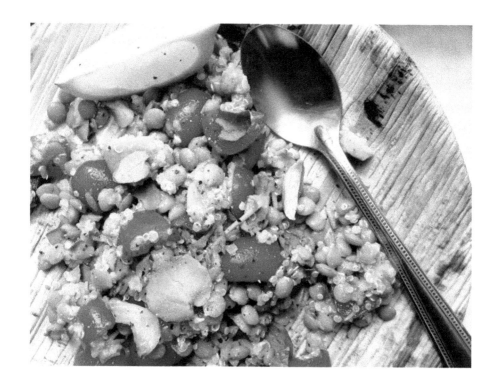

Cuban Beans and Rice

Preparation Time: 10 minutes | Cooking Time: 55 minutes | Servings: 6

Ingredients:

- 1 cup uncooked white rice

- 1 green bell pepper, cored, chopped

- 15.25 ounces cooked kidney beans

- 1 cup chopped white onion

- 4 tablespoons tomato paste

- 1 teaspoon minced garlic

- 1 teaspoon salt

- 1 tablespoon olive oil

- 2 ½ cups vegetable broth

Directions:

• Take a saucepan, place it over medium heat, add oil, and when hot, add onion, garlic, and bell pepper and cook for 5 minutes until tender.

• Then stir in salt and tomatoes, switch heat to the low level and cook for 2 minutes.

• Then stir in rice and beans, pour in the broth, stir until mixed and cook for 45 minutes until rice has absorbed all the liquid.

• Serve straight away.

Nutrition:

Calories: 258 Cal | Fat: 3.2 g | Carbs: 49.3 g | Protein: 7.3 g | Fiber: 5 g

Brown Rice, Broccoli, and Walnut

Preparation Time: 5 minutes | Cooking Time: 18 minutes | Servings: 4

Ingredients:

- 1 cup of brown rice

- 1 medium white onion, peeled, chopped

- 1 pound broccoli florets

- ½ cup chopped walnuts, toasted

- ½ teaspoon minced garlic

- ⅛ teaspoon ground black pepper

- ½ teaspoon salt

- 1 tablespoon vegan butter

- 1 cup vegetable broth

- 1 cup shredded vegan cheddar cheese

Directions:

• Take a saucepan, place it over medium heat, add butter and when it melts, add onion and garlic and cook for 3 minutes.

• Stir in rice, pour in the broth, bring the mixture to boil, then switch heat to medium-low level and simmer until rice has absorbed all the liquid.

• Meanwhile, take a casserole dish, place broccoli florets in it, sprinkle with salt and black pepper, cover with a plastic wrap, and microwave for 5 minutes until tender.

• Place cooked rice in a dish, top with broccoli, sprinkle with nuts and cheese, and then serve.

Nutrition:

Calories: 368 Cal | Fat: 23 g | Carbs: 30.4 g | Protein: 15.1 g | Fiber: 5.7 g

Pecan Rice

Preparation Time: 5 minutes | Cooking Time: 10 minutes | Servings: 4

Ingredients:

- 1/4 cup chopped white onion

- 1/4 teaspoon ground ginger

- 1/2 cup chopped pecans

- 1/4 teaspoon salt

- 2 tablespoons minced parsley

- 1/4 teaspoon ground black pepper

- 1/4 teaspoon dried basil

- 2 tablespoons vegan margarine

- 1 cup brown rice, cooked

Directions:

• Take a skillet pan, place it over medium heat, add margarine and when it melts, add all the ingredients except for rice and stir until mixed.

• Cook for 5 minutes, then stir in rice until combined and continue cooking for 2 minutes.

• Serve straight away.

Nutrition:

Calories: 280 Cal | Fat: 16.1 g | Carbs: 31 g | Protein: 4.3 g | Fiber: 3.8 g

Broccoli and Rice Stir Fry

Preparation Time: 5 minutes | Cooking Time: 10 minutes | Servings: 8

Ingredients:

- 16 ounces frozen broccoli florets, thawed

- 3 green onions, diced

- ½ teaspoon salt

- ¼ teaspoon ground black pepper

- 2 tablespoons soy sauce

- 1 tablespoon olive oil

- 1 ½ cups white rice, cooked

Directions:

- Take a skillet pan, place it over medium heat, add broccoli, and cook for 5 minutes until tender-crisp.

- Then add scallion and other ingredients, toss until well mixed, and cook for 2 minutes until hot.

- Serve straight away.

Nutrition:

Calories: 187 Cal | Fat: 3.4 g | Carbs: 33 g | Protein: 6.3 g | Fiber: 2.3 g

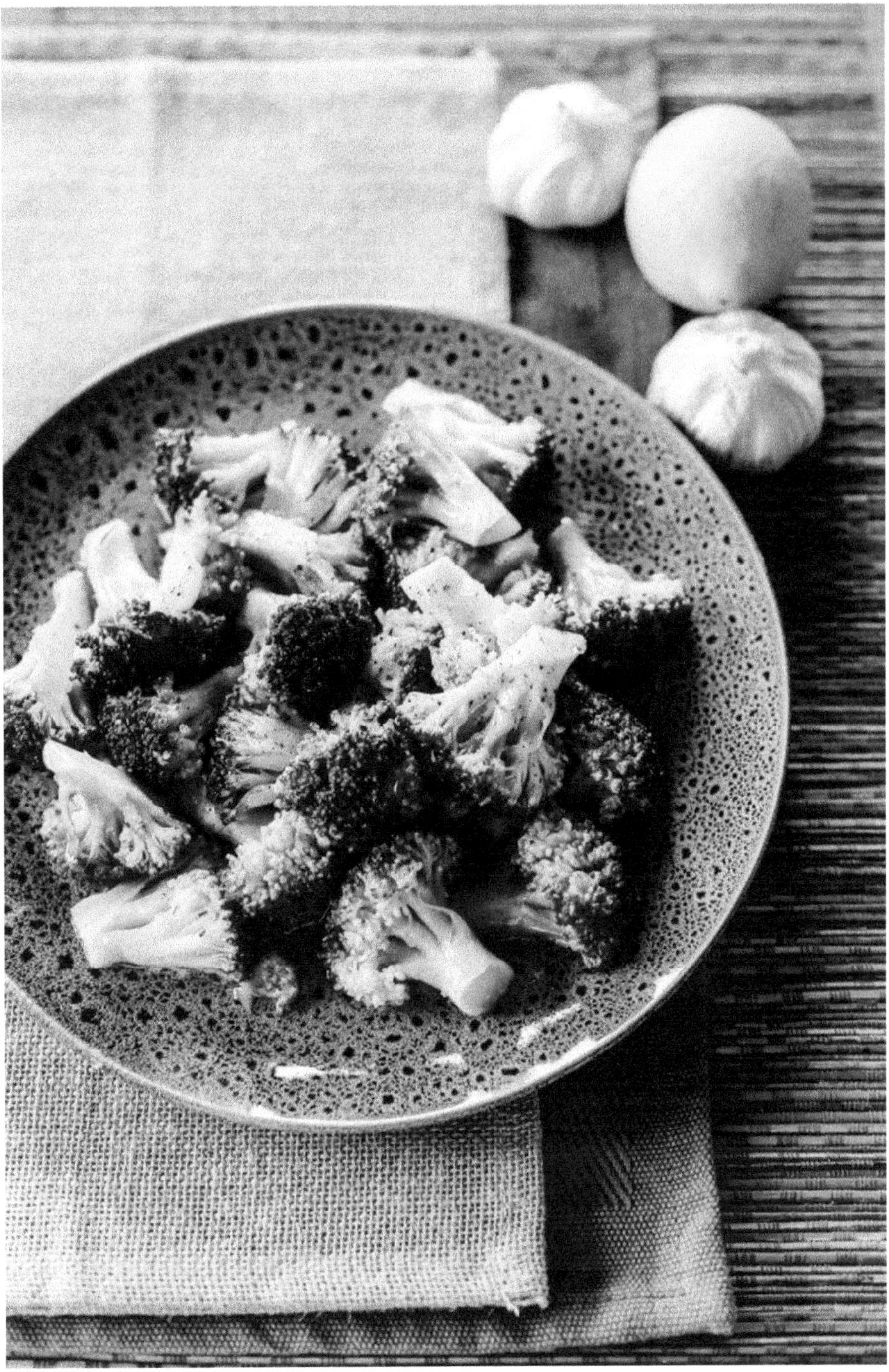

Lightning Source UK Ltd.
Milton Keynes UK
UKHW020757030621
384857UK00005B/84

9 781802 776645